Living with

Diabetes

Living with Series #5

HOW TO BE DIABETES FREE

By:

Kevin R. Sweeter

Contents

Aromatherapy

Meditation

Music and Sounds

Exercise and Physical Activity

Visual Aides

Hobbies and Distractions

Humor and Laughter

Social Interaction

Natural Surroundings

Sensory Deprivation / Overload

Introduction

Di·a·be·tes (dīə'bēdēz, dīə'bēdis) (**noun**) or **Hyperglycemia**

A disease in which the body's ability to produce or respond to the hormone insulin is impaired, resulting in abnormal metabolism of carbohydrates and elevated levels of glucose in the blood and urine.

Diabetes is a disease that affects your body's ability to produce or use insulin.

When your body turns the food you eat into energy, also called sugar or glucose, insulin is released to help transport this energy to the cells.

Insulin acts much like a key, where it sends a chemical message which tells the cell to open and receive glucose. If you produce little or no insulin, or are insulin resistant, and too much sugar remains in your blood.

Blood glucose levels are higher than normal for individuals with diabetes.

Myself, a diabetic for a number of years experienced the complications associated with diabetes, and these caused impairments that were getting intolerable. Medications were not addressing problem, and often carried undesirable side-effects.

With diligence, I embarked upon a quest to reverse the diabetic effects and eliminate the complications it was causing me. In a span of just a few months, I learned how to restore near-full function, and eliminated the majority of the problems.

My efforts continue, and my health improves daily. But, it requires a very strict discipline that you must learn to adhere to.

As anyone can tell you, before you can answer a question or arrive at an answer, you must first fully understand the question or the problem.

Let's embark now on the basics of the problem and get to understand what diabetes really is, then we will move on to what diabetes can and will do to you, and finally, I will offer you some solutions in how to deal with diabetes.

The first step, is to avoid getting diabetes in the first place. If you have a family history of diabetes, chances are likely that you will contract it, UNLESS you learn about what causes it. If you already have diabetes, then what you will learn here will help you fix that problem.

Diabetes Types

There are two main types of diabetes, or diabetes mellitus, Type 1 and Type 2.

Type 1 diabetes is also called juvenile diabetes, since it is often diagnosed in children or teens. This type accounts for 5-10 percent of people with diabetes.

When you are affected with Type 1 diabetes, your pancreas does not produce insulin. This is also referred to as **Maturity Onset Diabetes of the Young**

Type 2 diabetes occurs when the body does not produce enough insulin, or when the cells are unable to use insulin properly, which is called insulin resistance.

Type 2 diabetes is commonly called **Adult-Onset Diabetes**, or **Latent Autoimmune Diabetes in Adults**, since it is diagnosed later in life, generally after the age of 45, but can develop sooner.

Some 90 to 95 percent of people with diabetes have this type. In recent years, Type 2 diabetes has been diagnosed in younger people, including children, more frequently than in the past.

Gestational diabetes occurs during pregnancy and affects about 18 percent of all pregnancies, according to the American Diabetes Association.

Gestational diabetes usually goes away after pregnancy, but once you've had gestational diabetes, your chances are higher that it will happen in future pregnancies. In some women, pregnancy uncovers a predilection towards Type 1 or Type 2 diabetes, and these women will need to continue diabetes treatment after pregnancy.

There seems to be a link between the tendency to have gestational diabetes and Type 2 diabetes, and many women who had gestational diabetes develop Type 2 diabetes later on.

Gestational diabetes and Type 2 diabetes both involve insulin resistance. Certain basic lifestyle changes may help prevent diabetes after gestational diabetes.

Pre-diabetes is a condition that causes a person's blood sugar levels to be higher than normal but not high enough to be diagnosed with diabetes.

The American Diabetes Association estimates that there are 41 million Americans that have pre-diabetes in addition to the 18.2 million with diabetes.

Now consider, if your body has a difficulty either producing or using insulin, the problem is that your body cannot handle or process sugars. You can reduce your risk of diabetes by avoiding consumption of sugars and alcohol. Alcohol breaks down directly into sugars once the liver has processed it. This is what the liver does, it produces glucose for your body, and if it is functioning as it should, it will provide you with all the glucose your body will ever need.

Hypoglycemia, or low blood sugar / glucose

When blood glucose levels drop below normal levels, it is called **Hypoglycemia**.

The onset of hypoglycemia can be immediate with a variety of symptoms:

Clumsiness (more than usual)

Ataxia, incoordination, (resembling a drunken condition)

Difficulty speaking

Shakiness

Anxiety

Tachycardia

Sweating

A warm feeling

Pallor

Coldness, or Clamminess

Dilated pupils

Hunger

Nausea, vomiting, or abdominal discomfort

Headaches

Confusion

Light headedness, or dizziness

Abnormal thinking

Impaired judgment

Nonspecific dysphoria

Moodiness

Depressing

Crying

Stupor

Abnormal breathing

Exaggerated concerns

Numbness, or sensations of pins and needles

Loss of consciousness

Personality changes, or emotional liability

Fatigue, or weakness, or lethargy

Memory loss

Delirium

Glassy look, or staring

Blurred or double vision

Flashes of light in your field of vision

Automatism, or automatic behavior

Seizures, generalized or focal

Coma

Focal or generalized motor deficit, paralysis, or hemiparesis

and death.

Not all of these can or will occur and there seems to be no consistent order or pattern to the appearance of such symptoms, if any occur at all.

As with the varied symptoms described as non predictable, age can easily effect different symptoms as well. A younger child may vomit, whereas an older child may show signs is mania or a mental illness. Even in the same individual, the symptoms can vary greatly.

Symptoms can also manifest themselves as an individual sleeps. Having nightmares or crying out can be signs of hypoglycemia as well as bed sweating. Upon waking, the individual may seem irritable, confused, or feel tired.

Often, hypoglycemia won't cause long-term difficulties if addressed in time, and even if severe enough to cause unconsciousness or seizures, there is little risk of damaging the brain.

Death is a result of prolonged and untreated unconsciousness, interference with breathing, severe concurrent disease, or some other vulnerability.

Many of the described symptoms can have other legitimate causes, so the diagnosis of hypoglycemia may not be all that straightforward.

One indicator is if sugars are introduced into the system do not reverse the hypoglycemic condition after ten to 15 minutes, then another cause is most likely.

Long-term hypoglycemic effects can have negative impacts upon cardiovascular systems, and cause cardiovascular disease or at least contribute to the development.

General causes:

Hypoglycemia is often caused by a reaction to insulin medications, sepsis, kidney failure, some tumors, and liver disease (when the liver is not producing enough glucose), hypothyroidism, starvation, inborn error of metabolism, severe infections, reactive hypoglycemia, and a number of medications used to treat hyperglycemia (high).

This condition can also occur in healthy babies who have not eaten for a few hours.

The risk is greater in diabetics who have not eaten enough, or recently enough, have exercised more than usual, or have developed kidney or liver problems.

This can be a temporary condition in diabetics, but it is a very serious one, as it can result in death if not corrected immediately.

Diabetics can often experience these symptoms when fasting.

Normal glucose levels range typically from 70 mg/dL to 100 mg/ dL, (milligrams per deciliter) whereas you are considered hypoglycemic if glucose levels drop below this, and hyperglycemic if they exceed this range.

To remedy the hypoglycemic (low) levels, consumption of simple sugars such as found in a sugar laden food, or fruit juices.

Common Causes / Symptoms and Signs of Hyperglycemia (high blood sugar)

The actual cause of diabetes is unknown. Genetics, diet, obesity, and lack of exercise may play a role in developing diabetes, especially with Type 2 diabetes.

The causes that trigger diabetes type 1 and the process of self-destruction of the insulin-producing Beta cells are still unknown.

The disease begins when the already 80 to 90% of the cells are destroyed without showing any symptoms earlier.

There are too many types of diabetes that, even if it comes in a different form, the result is always the loss of the ability to produce insulin.

Diabetes type 1 or insulin dependent diabetes may develop due to disease of the pancreas, infectious or traumatic events like car accidents or surgery, but more often, it becomes the first type of diabetes without being affected by such events.

The disease usually affects children in childhood or adolescence, but there are cases of adults who develop this form after thirty years of age.

The adult form of diabetes can develop in individuals who are overweight or obese. This form is not manifested in a sharp contrast to the juvenile diabetes but rather gradually, often characterized by mild hyperglycemia, a slow onset, but steady.

In this case, insulin production doesn't cease immediately but also gradually, both possibly attributable to the huge presence of fat and sugar caused by incorrect or out of control diets, from periods of very heavy stress that put a strain on the mental and physical strength of an individual.

Insulin production becomes insufficient to compensate for the overwhelming amounts of sugars in the system.

Consequently, insulin production decreases until it ceased entirely, and this condition also contributes greatly to the occurrence of heart attacks and sclerosis.

This is a diabetes type that should not be underestimated, because it acts without obvious symptoms until it manifests itself through a traumatic event such as stroke.

In order to identify it, you need to do a simple blood test.

Contrarily to the other two forms of Diabetes, gestational diabetes occurs in some women during pregnancy, in particularly in those women who are overweight.

This type is not permanent, but may be indicative of a possible onset of diabetes type 2 during the menopause sometime in a woman's future.

Gestational diabetes arises from a temporary pressure on the insulin-producing cells during pregnancy and can't meet the needs required.

The classical symptoms of diabetes are polyuria, or frequent urination, polydipsia, or increased thirst, polyphagia, or increased hunger, blurred vision, fatigue, numbness or tingling in the hands or feet, sores that do not heal, and unexplained weight loss.

Symptoms of type 1 diabetes can start quickly, in a matter of weeks. Symptoms of type 2 diabetes often develop slowly, over the course of several years, and can be so mild that you might not even notice them.

Many people with type 2 diabetes have no symptoms at all and often do not find out they have the disease until they have diabetes-related health problems, such as blurred vision or heart trouble.

As in type 1 diabetes, certain genes may make you more likely to develop type 2 diabetes. The disease tends to run in families and occurs more often in these racial or ethnic groups:

African Americans

Alaska Natives

American Indians

Asian Americans

Hispanics/Latinos

Native Hawaiians

Pacific Islanders

Cushing's syndrome occurs when the body produces too much cortisol, often called the stress hormone.

Acromegaly occurs when the body produces too much growth hormone.

Hyperthyroidism occurs when the thyroid gland produces too much thyroid hormone.

Pancreatitis, pancreatic cancer, and trauma can all harm the beta cells or make them less able to produce insulin, resulting in diabetes.

If the damaged pancreas is removed, diabetes will occur due to the loss of the beta cells.

Sometimes certain medicines can harm beta cells or disrupt the way insulin works.

These include:

Niacin, a type of vitamin B3

Certain types of diuretics, also called water pills

Anti-seizure drugs

Psychiatric drugs

Drugs to treat human immunodeficiency virus (HIV)

Pentamidine, a drug used to treat a type of pneumonia

Glucocorticoids, medicines used to treat inflammatory illnesses such as rheumatoid arthritis, asthma, lupus, and ulcerative colitis

Anti-rejection medicines, used to help stop the body from rejecting a transplanted organ

Statins, which are medicines to reduce LDL, or bad, cholesterol levels, can slightly increase the chance that you'll develop diabetes.

However, statins help protect you from heart disease and stroke. For this reason, the strong benefits of taking statins outweigh the small chance that you could develop diabetes.

I firmly believe that I managed to manifest my onset on diabetes due directly to my poor eating habits. I consumed far too much sugar in my diet, caffeine levels that should have killed a Rhino, and far too much fast food.

Had I known earlier that my path was going to be this destructive, I would have been far more moderate in consuming these foods, and may have prevented the onset entirely. Lessons learned that I am now passing onto you.

Side effects and Health Concerns

After you eat or drink, your body breaks down the sugars in your blood and turns it into glucose. The glucose travels through your bloodstream and provides your body with energy.

To accomplish this, your pancreas needs to produce a hormone called insulin. In a person with diabetes, also diabetes mellitus, the pancreas either produces too little insulin or none at all, or the insulin can't be used effectively.

This allows blood glucose levels to rise while the rest of your cells are deprived of much needed energy. This can lead to a wide variety of problems affecting nearly every part of your body.

The main problem in Type 2 diabetes is the presence of what is called insulin resistance. In this sort of diabetes, the pancreas starts off robust in its production of insulin.

However, cells that need energy don't respond normally to the usual amounts of insulin. The pancreas has to produce much higher levels of the hormone in order to manage blood glucose levels.

Over time, the insulin-producing cells in the pancreas can burn themselves out due to this overproduction. At this point, a person with Type 2 diabetes begins to require insulin medication.

However, in earlier phases of this more common type of diabetes, the illness can be effectively managed with diet, exercise, and careful monitoring of blood sugars.

Some people with Type 2 diabetes may require a variety of oral medications and eventually, as described above, some will eventually need insulin.

Gestational diabetes is high blood sugar that develops during pregnancy. Most of the time, gestational diabetes can be controlled through diet and exercise, and it typically resolves after the baby is delivered.

Endocrine, Excretory, and Digestive Systems

Your pancreas produces and releases insulin to help make energy out of sugars. If your pancreas produces little or no insulin, or if your body can't use it, alternate hormones are used to turn fat into energy.

This can create high levels of toxic chemicals, including acids and ketone bodies, which may lead to a condition called diabetic ketoacidosis.

This is a serious complication of the disease. Symptoms include extreme thirst, excessive urination, and fatigue. Your breath may have a sweet scent that is caused by the elevated levels of ketone bodies in the blood.

High blood sugar levels and excess ketones in your urine can confirm diabetic ketoacidosis. Untreated, the condition can lead to loss of consciousness or even death.

Diabetes can damage your kidneys, affecting their ability to filter waste products from your blood.

Elevated amounts of protein in your urine, micro albuminuria, may be a sign that your kidneys aren't functioning properly. Kidney disease related to diabetes is called diabetic nephropathy.

This condition doesn't show symptoms until it advances to later stages. People with diabetes should be evaluated for nephropathy in order to avoid irreversible kidney damage and kidney failure.

Diabetic hyperglycemic hyperosmolar syndrome occurs in Type 2 diabetes.

It involves very high blood glucose levels but without ketones. Symptoms also include dehydration and loss of consciousness.

It usually happens to people whose diabetes is undiagnosed or who have not been able to control their diabetes. It can also be caused by heart attack, stroke, or infection.

High blood glucose levels can make it hard for your stomach to completely empty, gastro paresis.

In turn, the delay causes blood glucose levels to rise.

Diabetes is the leading cause of gastro paresis. Symptoms include nausea, vomiting, bloating, and heartburn.

Circulatory System

High blood glucose levels can contribute to the formation of fatty deposits in blood vessel walls. Over time, that can restrict blood flow and increase the risk of hardening of the blood vessels, atherosclerosis.

Lack of blood flow can affect your hands and feet. Poor circulation can cause pain in the calves while you're walking, intermittent claudication.

People with diabetes are particularly prone to foot problems due to narrowed blood vessels in the leg and foot.

Your feet may feel cold, and you may be unable to feel heat due to lack of sensation.

A condition called diabetic neuropathy causes decreased sensation in the extremities, which may prevent you from noticing an injury or infection.

Diabetes increases your risk of developing infections or ulcers of the foot. Poor blood flow and nerve damage increase the likelihood of having a foot or leg amputated.

If you have diabetes, it is critical that you take good care of your feet and inspect them often.

Diabetes raises your risk of developing high blood pressure, putting strain on the heart. According to the National Diabetes Information Clearinghouse, people with diabetes have double the risk of heart disease or stroke than people without diabetes.

Monitoring and controlling your blood glucose, blood pressure, and cholesterol can lower that risk. So can good eating habits and exercise.

Diabetes and smoking are a very bad mix, increasing risk of cardiovascular problems and restricted blood flow.

Integumentary System

Diabetes can affect your skin. Lack of moisture can cause the skin on your feet to dry and crack. It is important to completely dry your feet after bathing or swimming.

You can use petroleum jelly or gentle creams, but be careful as creams or oils left between your toes can become so moist that it can lead to infection.

High-pressure spots under your foot can lead to calluses.

If you don't take good care of them, they can become infected or develop ulcers. If you get an ulcer, see your doctor immediately to lower your risk of losing your foot.

You may also be more prone to boils, infection of the hair follicles, folliculitis, sties, and infected nails. People with diabetes have a higher incidence of bacterial infections, including staph, or Staphylococcus, than the general population.

Moist, warm folds in the skin are susceptible to fungal or yeast infections. You're most likely to develop this type of infection between fingers and toes, the groin, armpits, or in the corners of your mouth.

Symptoms include redness, blistering, and itchiness.

A condition called diabetic dermopathy can cause brown patches on the skin. There's no cause for concern and no treatment is necessary.

Eruptive xanthomatosis causes hard yellow bumps with a red ring. Digital sclerosis causes thick skin, most often on the hands or feet. Both of these skin conditions are signs of unmanaged diabetes.

They usually clear up when you get your blood sugar under control.

Central Nervous System

Diabetes causes damage to the nerves, also known as peripheral neuropathy, which can affect your perception of heat, cold, and pain, making you more susceptible to injury.

This also makes it more likely that you'll ignore an injury, especially if it's in a difficult place to see, such as between your toes, on your heels, or the bottoms of your feet.

Swollen, leaky blood vessels in the eye, diabetic retinopathy, can damage your vision and even lead to blindness.

Symptoms include floaters or spots in your field of vision. People with diabetes tend to develop cataracts at an earlier age than other people.

They are also more likely to develop glaucoma.

Symptoms of eye trouble can be mild at first, so it's important to see your eye doctor regularly.

Reproductive System

The hormones of pregnancy can cause gestational diabetes. This also increases the risk of high blood pressure, preeclampsia, or ecclampsia.

In most cases, gestational diabetes is easily controlled, and glucose levels return to normal after the baby is born.

Symptoms are the same as other types of diabetes, but may also include repeated infections affecting the vagina and bladder.

Women with gestational diabetes may have babies with higher birth weight, making delivery more complicated. Women who have had gestational diabetes should be monitored, as there's an increased risk of developing diabetes within ten years.

Erectile dysfunction

Diabetes is probably the number one cause of erectile dysfunction, and will impair your sex drive and life. This is not something men would ever choose to have as an affliction or side effect of any physical condition.

Ocular impairment

Prolonged elevated blood glucose levels will eventually begin to affect and impair visual acuity, cause damage to the blood vessels in the eye by affecting blood pressure levels, and promote degradation of the macula, which can lead to eventual loss of sight.

Balance control issues

Elevated glucose levels can have detrimental effects on your ability to balance while standing or walking, and this can lead to tendencies of falling, tripping, and other potential injury causing incidents. It may also eventually require the use of walking aides such as a cane, walker, or eventually even become wheelchair bound.

Loss of motor control

Along with balance control issues, you may begin to ind issues with controlling your muscular structure. Grip strength is often the first to be noticeably affected, or the potential for random and sudden loss of grip, thus causing you to drop objects from your hands. Knee buckling is another random malfunction that can easily surprise you at any point and possibly cause a fall of some sort, or a misstep leading to the same potential physical injury.

Essential Tremors

Typically, tremors that develop as a result of diabetes is generally attributed to the consumption of artificial sweetening agents, but can happen with any sugar consumption. Especially drinking quantities of soda or candies will inevitably result in shaking hands. Not only is this rather embarrassing to live with in public, but it will also impair you from performing even the most simple functions in life. Holding food on a fork becomes an impossible challenge, not to mention attempting to perform any intricate task, like threading a small screw into a slot, or threading a sewing needle, or tying a shoelace will become frustratingly difficult.

Renal Failure or complications

Kidney failure or complications are no laughing matter, and is a very serious health condition and unless treated immediately, death is often eminent. You will slowly poison yourself without the kidneys functioning properly.

Kidney dialysis is an artificial, mechanical method and procedure used to detoxify the blood in the body by

removing waste, salts, and extra water from the body to prevent build up. It also helps to stabilize certain chemicals in the blood to stable and healthy levels, such as potassium, sodium, and bicarbonate. It can also help to stabilize blood pressure.

There are two types of dialysis: hemodialysis and peritoneal dialysis.

Hemodialysis

In hemodialysis, an artificial kidney (hemodialyzer) is used to remove waste and extra chemicals and fluid from your blood. To get your blood into the artificial kidney, the doctor needs to make an access (entrance) into your blood vessels. This is done by minor surgery to your arm or leg.

Sometimes, an access is made by joining an artery to a vein under your skin to make a bigger blood vessel called a fistula.

However, if your blood vessels are not adequate for a fistula, the doctor may use a soft plastic tube to join an artery and a vein under your skin. This is called a graft.

Occasionally, an access is made by means of a narrow plastic tube, called a catheter, which is inserted into a large vein in your neck. This type of access may be temporary, but is sometimes used for long-term treatment.

The time needed for your dialysis depends on:

• how well your kidneys work

• how much fluid weight you gain between treatments

• how much waste you have in your body

• how big you are

• the type of artificial kidney used

Usually, each hemodialysis treatment lasts about four hours and is done three times per week.

A type of hemodialysis called high-flux dialysis may take less time. You can speak to your doctor to see if this is an appropriate treatment for you.

Peritoneal dialysis

In this type of dialysis, your blood is cleaned inside your body. The doctor will do surgery to place a plastic tube called a catheter into your abdomen (belly) to make an access. During the treatment, your abdominal area (called the peritoneal cavity) is slowly filled with dialysate through the catheter. The blood stays in the arteries and veins that line your peritoneal cavity. Extra fluid and waste products are drawn out of your blood and into the dialysate. There are two major kinds of peritoneal dialysis.

What are the different kinds of peritoneal dialysis and how do they work?

There are several kinds of peritoneal dialysis but two major ones are:

Continuous Ambulatory Peritoneal Dialysis (CAPD) and Automated Peritoneal Dialysis (APD)

Continuous Ambulatory Peritoneal Dialysis (CAPD) is the only type of peritoneal dialysis that is done without machines. You do this yourself, usually four, or five times a day at home and/or at work. You put a bag of dialysate, usually about two quarts, into your peritoneal cavity through the catheter. The dialysate stays there for about four or five hours before it is drained back into the bag and thrown away. This is called an exchange. You use a new bag of dialysate each time you do an exchange. While the dialysate is in your peritoneal cavity, you can go about your usual activities at work, at school or at home.

Automated Peritoneal Dialysis (APD) usually is done at home using a special machine called a cycler. This is similar to CAPD except that a number of cycles or exchanges, occur. Each cycle usually lasts 1-1/2 hours and exchanges are done throughout the night while you sleep.

Dialysis can be done in a hospital, in a dialysis unit that is not part of a hospital, or at home. You and your doctor will decide which place is best, based on your medical condition and your wishes.

Dialysis does some of the work of healthy kidneys, but it does not cure your kidney disease. You will need to have dialysis treatments for your whole life unless you are able to get a kidney transplant.

You may have some discomfort when the needles are put into your fistula or graft, but most patients have no other problems. The dialysis treatment itself is painless.

However, some patients may have a drop in their blood pressure. If this happens, you may feel sick to your stomach, vomit, have a headache or cramps. With frequent treatments, those problems usually go away.

Hemodialysis and peritoneal dialysis have been done since the mid 1940s. Dialysis, as a regular treatment, began in 1960 and is now a standard treatment all around the world. CAPD began in 1976. Thousands of patients have been helped by these treatments.

If your kidneys have failed, you will need to have dialysis treatments for your whole life unless you are able to get a kidney transplant. Life expectancy on dialysis can vary depending on your other medical conditions and how well you follow your treatment plan. Average life expectancy on dialysis is 5-10 years, however, many patients have lived well on dialysis for 20 or even 30 years. Talk to your healthcare team about how to take care of yourself and stay healthy on dialysis.

Dialysis costs a lot of money. However, the federal government pays 80 percent of all dialysis costs for most patients. Private health insurance or state Medicaid programs also help with the costs.

Many patients live normal lives except for the time needed for treatments. Dialysis usually makes you feel better because it helps many of the problems caused by kidney failure. You and your family will need time to get used to dialysis.

You may be on a special diet. You may not be able to eat everything you like, and you may need to limit how much you drink. Your diet may vary according to the type of dialysis.

Dialysis centers are located in every part of the United States and in many foreign countries. The treatment is standardized. You must make an appointment for dialysis treatments at another center before you go. The staff at your center may help you make the appointment.

Many dialysis patients can go back to work after they have gotten used to dialysis. If your job has a lot of physical labor (heavy lifting, digging, etc...), you may need to get a different job.

Kidney failure is permanent

It usually is, but not always. Some kinds of acute kidney failure get better after treatment. In some cases of acute kidney failure, dialysis may only be needed for a short time until the kidneys get better.

In chronic or end stage kidney failure, your kidneys do not get better and you will need dialysis for the rest of your life. If your doctor says you are a candidate, you may choose to be placed on a waiting list for a new kidney.

These are but a few of the potential complications that will almost certainly affect all diabetics at some point unless they decide to try to improve the situation.

Unchecked, diabetes will only lead to complications from issues resulting from the diabetes, the added burden of mobility issues not only upon the diabetic, but also friends and family members who are called upon to assist the diabetic though life.

How is Diabetes Diagnosed?

Out of the estimated 24 million people with diabetes, one third, or eight million, don't even know they have the disease because people with type 2 diabetes often have no symptoms.

However, a simple blood test is all you need to find out if you are one the millions with untreated diabetes.

The American Diabetes Association (ADA) recommends that everyone aged 45 and over should be tested for diabetes, and if the results are normal, re-tested every three years.

Testing should be conducted at earlier ages and carried out more frequently in individuals who have any of the following diabetes risk factors:

You have a parent or sibling with diabetes

You are overweight, with a BMI higher than 25

You are a member of a high-risk ethnic population

You had gestational diabetes or a baby weighing over 9 pounds

Your HDL cholesterol levels are 35 mg/dl or less, and/or your triglyceride level is 250 mg/dl or above

You have high blood pressure

You have polycystic ovarian syndrome

On previous testing, you had impaired glucose tolerance or impaired fasting tolerance

Fasting Plasma Glucose

This blood test is taken in the morning, on an empty stomach. A level of 126 mg/dl or above, on more than one occasion, indicates diabetes.

Casual or Random Glucose

This blood test can be taken anytime during the day, without fasting. A glucose level of 200 mg/dl and above may suggest diabetes.

If any of these test results occurs, testing should be repeated on a different day to confirm the diagnosis. If a casual plasma glucose equal to 200 mg/dl or above is detected, the confirming test used should be a fasting plasma glucose or an oral glucose tolerance test.

Food Pharmacy - Eating your way to a Diabetes-Free life

As the old saying goes, 'You are what you eat'. This also goes with how, and what you feel like each day.

It is little known that certain foods, which when consumed, can cause emotional responses, or reactions, good and bad.

For diabetics, this situation is unique and not understood by the general or mainstream medical industry and dietitians.

Through ignorance or misinformation, physicians in general, and dietitians on the whole do NOT know how or what a Diabetic should eat.

Understand the problem of a diabetic.

Diabetics already have a problem processing sugars in their bodies. This means that any sugars introduced into the body will not be dealt with by the body, and thus remain in the blood stream as excess glucose.

The human body is protein based, and I don't care how long or hard a vegan will argue this point, but it is a simple, biological fact.

Without proteins, the body cannot function properly, build or maintain muscles, or heal properly.

True enough, some of the highest protein sources are indeed found in some vegetables, such as spinach, but please read on…

Carbohydrates ingested must be converted to sugars before the body can utilize them. Now, since diabetics already have a problem dealing with sugars, the body is not benefitting from consuming any carbohydrates.

Starches are worse than carbohydrates to a diabetic, as are grains and alcohols.

So, what should diabetics eat then?

Meats.

Plain and simple, unprocessed, un-breaded meats.

Processed meats are not good for anyone, and there is quite a list of these in markets all over the world today. It is rather difficult to find unprocessed meats.

Bacon, sausages, meats found in loaf forms (luncheon meats), chicken nuggets, fish sticks, and the like are all processed meats. Technically, ground beef by definition is a processed meat, but if organically produced would be an acceptable form.

Fish is a good source of proteins if you can manage an non-toxic source of seafood's. NEVER buy seafood of any sort that is 'FARM RAISED' especially from Asia. The Internet is replete with videos showing just how these 'farm raised' products are indeed raised, and frankly, the environment (especially China) is toxic. Try to source fresh caught seafood, this does make it rather difficult, but not impossible. Specialty stores will have a better source of seafood, however, mainstream food outlets will typically be getting their products from questionable sources.

Since we really cannot subsist entirely on just meats, I have found that organic protein powders help a great deal. It tends to be expensive, as does organic meats, (or any organic foods in general) but for your health, it is worth it.

Protein powders are typically mixed in water or milk, and whereas milk itself contains carbohydrates and sugars, it is easier to drink protein powders with milk than water for shear flavor purposes. If you are able to use strictly water, then by all means do so.

By switching my diet to meats, and protein powders, I was able to return my typical glucose levels to normal 70-100 range even after eating.

Eggs are an excellent source of protein with few carbohydrates included. However, it will be important to know how to prepare them for consumption. Be wary of using oils for frying eggs, as oils have a definite – and short-lived actual shelf life, and can easily add to the carbohydrate levels, and even starches to your foods. I boil eggs to be safe from adding anything to them.

Cheese is also a good source of proteins, however, most cheeses have an elevated saturated fat content, and we really shouldn't be adding the bad fats to our diet either. Different cheeses will have different levels of protein, and fat, but still keep the carbs down to a minimum.

Here are the rules:

These are very strict rules, and if you want to stop the damages caused by diabetes, and reverse the effects entirely you must adhere to them.

No Carbohydrates.

Or as few as possible. This means no vegetables, no fruits, no breads, no breaded meats, no gravies, no dressings. Even some condiments have something in them that is bad for you. I have found that mustard is relatively safe, as are most hot sauces.

No Sugars:

This means ALL sugars, natural or otherwise, and especially no artificial sweeteners. Companies have created 'diabetic' friendly 'diet' versions of soda, and other foods, but this is horribly misleading. These products use substances that are far worse for consumption than any natural sugar could ever be for anyone. (See my book on Toxic Foods). If your liver is functioning properly, it will provide your body with whatever amounts of glucose it requires. I have experimented with this extensively.

My research has shown that even during a starvation diet (that is consuming nothing more than plain tap water) I was maintaining higher levels of blood glucose than normal. This meant that my liver was delivering glucose to my blood at above-normal levels to compensate for the lack of ingested foods.

It is important to give your body what it needs in order to function, repair, and maintain itself in a healthy manner. Moderation in all things is the best way regardless. But nutrition is still very important.

Vitamin supplements such as C and E, may be needed when you feel ill or have some sort of damage to your body, calcium is important for maintaining bones and teeth. B complex vitamins will help with digestion, and so on.

If you eat anything, eat reduced portions. Never stuff yourself, and yes this also means especially during the holiday feast seasons where it is so tempting to eat your fill for even a couple of meals.

If you find yourself hungry, eat the smaller portions more frequently during the day. That old practice of eating three square meals per day is an antiquated practice that is not healthy for a diabetic to entertain anymore. Smaller, more controlled portions, over the entire day will help to keep glucose levels in your system at a stable and lower level generally. That is also the goal; to keep your glucose levels stable throughout the entire day, not rollercoaster them up and down with and between each meal.

Above all else, resist the temptation to eat anything not good for you, for even small portions of foods that contain carbohydrates and sugars (especially those that are high in these) will only serve to damage your body and reduce the chances that you can fix this problem.

It is probably impossible to eliminate all carbohydrates and sugars from your diet, but try your very best to reduce them all you can. Every little bit will add to the problem, and reducing every little bit will only help in the end.

Things to look for in the list of ingredients:

High Fructose corn syrup, Aspartame, sucrose, refined sugars. Even cane sugar is going to be bad for a diabetic.

Many foods, condiments, etc… have a lot of things added to them, READ THE LABELS. The longer the list of ingredients, the more processed the food will be.

No Starches

Starches are bad for even healthy people, and are rarely needed or utilized by the body. Yes, they can contribute to energy sometimes, but must be consumed in reduced quantities by healthy people to remain healthy. For a diabetic, they are disastrous. I love potatoes, but they are one of the worst types of foods for me as a diabetic.

No Grains

Breads, regardless of the grains (whole, or otherwise) are typically mostly carbohydrates and starches, with maybe some sugars included. The same can go for grains found in cereals (also all processed foods) and so called health foods like energy bars, and the like. ALL of these are bad for a diabetic. If you go out to eat, even an innocuous sandwich can have ill effects. If you must or are limited to foods available, get a burger without the bun or fixings. Yes, boring I know, but you can't have anything except the burger itself. Also, avoid mainstream brands of ketchup, which is usually made with toxic ingredients (as covered in my book titled 'Toxic Foods'), where I describe such bad ingredients.

Doctors and dietitians alike have recommended things like oatmeal for diabetics, and this is demonstrably wrong on their part. Oatmeal had high amounts of carbohydrates, and starches which your body cannot deal with properly.

Restaurants will gladly serve an entrée without the side dishes, and in most cases may even give you a slight break on the cost of the meal as a result. Ask them if they can discount part of your meal as a result of not getting the side dishes.

No Caffeine

Caffeine acts in the body as a sugar would; it readily and effectively increases blood glucose levels just as much as sugars and anything else will. So, that coffee with no cream or sugar in it thought to be safe for a diabetic to drink, is NOT safe to drink.

NO FAST FOODS

Fast foods are definitely **OFF** the menu forever. If you knew how much of that food is prepared, even not being diabetic, you would rather not eat any anyway – trust me.

This dietary change must happen gradually, or like with fad diets of all manner, your body will freak out and reject the attempt. Each time you eat, cut something bad for you out of the equation. I would eliminate sugars first off.

Secondly, begin to reduce and eliminate the grains and carbohydrates from your diet. It will get difficult, as we don't like to consume even a simple hamburger without the bun, or fixings. But you MUST eliminate these things from your diet. If you eat a hamburger, do not have the bread or the toppings along with it.

Yes, admittedly, your diet will get a little boring, but you will adapt if you stick with it. For diabetics who also suffer from Neuropathy, or Tremors, they will find almost immediate relief from these afflictions.

One possible undesirable side effect of consuming protein powders is that the body will generate ammonia during the conversion process. This is normal, but you will smell of ammonia when you perspire. This goes away once you stop perspiring.

There are many foods I do indeed miss eating, but they were causing harm to me by simply eating them. I was losing balance control and required things to help me walk and stand like a cane or a walker, I had terrible tremors, I had Neuropathy impairing my legs and hands, I was a wreck, and getting worse by the day.

All that began to change as soon as I cleaned up my diet.

Protein powder is going to be expensive, especially since you also have to source some that have no sweeteners included. I prefer an organic, grass-fed cow sourced protein with no hormones or GMOs involved.

Another issue with protein powder is that you have to mix it with something in order to consume it. Water is recommended, but very boring and quite honestly, tastes like crap! I do use organic milk, usually 1% to mix my protein in, and yes, milk has carbohydrates and sugars, but it is a slight setback that I am tolerant of because I subsist on this mostly over solid foods. Yet, I do maintain reasonable levels of glucose in my blood.

I recently discovered that there have been professional studies conducted in the UK which also confirm my own findings, where diet is indeed the key to curing diabetes.

Try it for a month at least; you will note the differences almost immediately. Ease into the new diet though, cut back where you can here and there, and reduce what bad foods you ingest, and increase the good stuff as you go. It is not easy to adapt to this practice, but the effects will amaze you in the end. As with all things, especially changes in lifestyle, you must adapt to it gradually. Also, it will help to reduce or eliminate the temptation of bad foods. Yes, this may not be easy if you live with people who are not diabetic, but if you don't have anything bad for you within reach or easy access, it will be easier to deal with those bad food cravings and avoid giving in to them if you can't actually find something to cheat with.

Above all else **<u>NO CHEATING</u>** , you cannot stray from this strict diet, or the effects will not go way entirely, or at all. Do not give in to temptation. If you have to, you must get rid of the bad stuff in the house, not having something around that you crave but is bad for you will go a long way in helping you stay on track.

It will be difficult, much like hanging out with friends who love to smoke or drink and you just gave those up. Eating is no different. Family can be unforgiving in this, and may not fully understand why or how you would need to give up most foods. Education is the key to success here, make them aware of the problem and the solution that must be managed, get them to help you stay on track with your strict regimen of meats, and proteins only diet. They will make things difficult by preparing and eating foods that smell so wonderful, and the temptation will be great.

I am thankful that I live where nobody will deliver anything as far as foods go, so there was no cheating when I couldn't drive anywhere by ordering a pizza or any other food bad for me. Isolation helped.

Good luck, and stick with it!

Trust that the little suffering you may endure with a new diet is far less painful and difficult than dealing with the loss of an extremity because your circulation was compromised by diabetes, or that you have to submit to kidney dialysis a few times each week, or that your mobility is impaired in any way requiring a cane, walker, or wheelchair.

If you yourself don't actually care about what happens to you, then that if your choice in life and nothing I can say will change that. But, if you live with someone who cares about you, loves you, or ends up having to care for you because you have lost that ability yourself, consider how much of a pain in the ass it will be for them to care for you, help you get around, and help you to do simple things you should be able to do on your own, but can't because you simply didn't care about your own health.

Herbs

There are herbs you can obtain that will help reduce glucose in your blood stream, but if you have corrected your diet effectively, then these would not even be needed. But when you are starting out trying to reduce your consumption of sugars and carbohydrates, these will contribute to your wellbeing.

I preferred to use herbal teas to help reduce glucose levels at first. They can be found at most health food stores or specialty tea web sites. The benefit of using tea reduces the intake of carbohydrates while obtaining the benefits of the effect of the herbs used.

Many of these teas may not taste good to many people, but it will be a necessary evil for at least a little while. If you find that they are tasty, all the better.

Aloe vera (/ˈæloʊiː/ or /ˈæloʊ/) is a plant species of the genus Aloe, which grows wild in tropical climates around the world and is cultivated for agricultural and medicinal uses.

Oral ingestion of aloe vera may cause abdominal cramps and diarrhea, which in turn can decrease the absorption of drugs.

Bilberry extract (Vaccinium myrtillus)

Vaccinium myrtillus is a species of shrub with edible fruit of blue color, commonly called 'bilberry', 'wimberry', 'whortleberry, or 'European blueberry'.

Vaccinium myrtillus has been used for nearly 1,000 years in traditional European medicine. Vaccinium myrtillus fruits have been used in the traditional Austrian medicine internally directly or as tea or liqueur, for treatment of disorders of the gastrointestinal tract and diabetes.

Herbal supplements of V. myrtillus on the market are used for circulatory problems, as vision aids, and to treat diarrhea and other conditions.

Bitter Melon (Momordica charantia)

Momordica charantia, known as 'bitter melon', 'bitter gourd', 'bitter squash', or 'balsam-pear', is a tropical and subtropical vine of the family Cucurbitaceae, widely grown in Asia, Africa, and the Caribbean for its edible fruit.

With regard to the use of Momordica charantia for diabetes, several animal studies and small-scale human studies have demonstrated a hypoglycemic effect of concentrated bitter melon extracts. Additionally, a 2014 review shows evidence that Momordica charantia, when consumed in raw or juice form, can be efficacious in lowering blood glucose levels.

Reported side effects include diarrhea, abdominal pain, fever, hypoglycemia, urinary incontinence, and chest pain. Symptoms are generally mild, and do not require treatment, often resolve themselves with rest.

Bitter melon is contraindicated in pregnant women because it can induce bleeding, contractions, and miscarriage.

Cinnamon (/ˈsɪnəmən/ SIN-ə-mən) is a spice obtained from the inner bark of several tree species from the genus Cinnamomum.

Cinnamon has a long history of use in traditional medicine. It has been tested in a variety of clinical conditions, such as bronchitis or diabetes, where it is believed to help reduce blood glucose levels. This has not yet been scientifically verified. However, it does add a pleasant flavor to many foods and beverages.

Fenugreek (/ˈfɛnjʊɡriːk/; Trigonella foenum-graecum) is an annual plant in the family Fabaceae.

Some people are allergic to fenugreek, and people who have peanut allergy and chickpea allergy may have a reaction to fenugreek.

Fenugreek seeds can cause diarrhea, dyspepsia, abdominal distention, flatulence, perspiration, and a maple-like smell to urine or breast milk.

There is a risk of hypoglycemia particularly in people with diabetes; it may also interfere with the activity of anti-diabetic drugs.

In traditional medicine, fenugreek is thought to promote digestion, induce labor, and reduce blood sugar levels in diabetics.

Ginger (Zingiber officinale) is a flowering plant whose rhizome, ginger root or simply ginger, is widely used as a spice, tea, or a folk medicine.

If consumed in reasonable quantities, ginger has few negative side effects though it does interact with some medications.

Allergic reactions to ginger generally result in a rash.

Okra, (US: /ˈoʊkrə/ or UK: /ˈɒkrə/), Abelmoschus esculentus is a flowering plant in the mallow family.

Medications for diabetes prescribed by physicians DO NOT address the problem of diabetes; they ONLY cause the blood glucose levels to drop. This is a short-term 'band-aide' so-called 'solution' to a more complicated problem that much be addressed properly in order to resolve the actual issues at hand.

Insulin is often prescribed to augment the insulin levels in the body. These may help the body utilize glucose to some degree, but it still does not address the actual issue.

Relaxation Techniques

The following outlined relaxation therapy methods are a great start to helping you deal with anything in life. If you can manage to calm yourself inwardly, and allow yourself to relax and reconnect with yourself, you are already well on your way to healing and recovery from just about anything in life.

Any one of these methods can be effective, but I would recommend using a combination of two or more if possible. As these are never harmful in any way, you cannot overdose or suffer ill effects from practicing them.

Keep in mind that with anything new in life, start off slow, gradually adapting to the new practices. It will make the transitions much more easily possible and effective.

Aromatherapy

The employment of pleasant aromas, odors, and smells.

It is a remarkable and effective practice to immerse yourself with something that smells very comforting or pleasant to you. It can be a simple smell, or a variety of them. Gardens, greenhouses, and other such locations can offer the pleasant aroma of flowers and plants. This may not always be suitable for those with allergies though.

Other sources are extracts you can get from most suppliers of health food products. Lavender, Mint, Pine, all can give you a sense of comfort by having them near you. Again, if allergies are a problem, then avoid this particular method entirely.

There are also scented candles, incense; even car air fresheners which can make a difference, provided the aromas produced are indeed pleasant.

Certain perfumes can have some powerful effects, both positively and negatively, so use caution. If a certain smell reminds you of a particularly bad date, relationship, or situation, well, avoid that.

The idea is to immerse yourself if you are able in an environment that invokes a pleasant experience. Pleasant is calming, soothing, relaxing, and comforting. All these will help to ease and reduce tensions, and things aggravating, upsetting, or any unpleasant condition you may be experiencing.

If allergies are not an issue, I would also recommend pairing this method up with Meditation.

Meditation

You have seen or are at least aware of meditation, usually promoted by the likes of Yoga enthusiasts, Buddha monks, etc... but you need not get all that elaborate in practice.

A simple and effective method of meditation merely requires a place of solitude, preferably a quiet, secluded spot, even if it is just a closet in your home, and usually low, or very soft lighting or even complete darkness.

How you sit is also important. You need to be comfortable, and also to be able to sit in the same position for a specific period of time.

If you need to adjust your position frequently, then you should work on that until you find a way to be able to remain motionless without cramping, pinching nerves, or causing any discomfort. The goal is to be comfortable, but not so much as you fall asleep.

When you have worked out your physical position, then begin with clearing your mind. Completely empty it of all thoughts, especially anything of negative origin.

Work on your breathing

Control your breath. Take in deep, deliberate breaths; take your time about it. Fill your lungs gradually to full capacity, hold at the maximum filled capacity for a moment or two, then release just as gradually and deliberately, not forcing, but letting it just slip out.

You may experience a slight dizziness while doing this, but that is because you are oversupplying oxygen to areas not regularly used to having so much. In time, you will be able to adapt to this sensation.

Repeat the breathing, all the while clearing your mind of all thoughts and processes. You can even just concentrate on the breathing exercise, counting seconds while breathing in, and then out again. This will help to clear the mind as well.

Eventually, slow your breathing further, no need to fully inflate your lungs so much, just return gradually to your normal breathing pattern.

You will feel a calmness settle in, your mind will be clear; your body will tingle slightly. You will relax more easily.

The length of time you meditate will depend entirely upon you. If you are exceptionally distressed, then more time may be needed. You should then also concentrate directly on calming yourself down, making yourself believe that all is well, that there is nothing to be afraid of, angry with, or distressed about. You are safe and secure. Nothing bad will happen.

If you are ill or injured, use this to 'command' your body to repair itself. This is not only possible, but the best possible way to heal. Your mind controls and directs the body. The body will obey. Oh, it may be stubborn at first, and not want to listen, but it will. You are in control, you make the decisions, you give the commands, they body must obey.

The great thing about meditation is that after you have practiced this enough, you can learn to adapt your meditation practice to everyday life and situations. Even while sitting at a desk at some place of work, you can practice the calming and breathing methods wherever you are. It may be more distracting in some places, but as with practice, eventually you could accomplish this regardless of where you are, even in the most noisy and public places. I would not recommend practicing this while operating any sort of machinery though, that would be potentially disastrous.

With the silence, you can also introduce music and sounds if you like.

Music and Sounds

Whatever you choose to listen to while meditating or even just unwinding, it should be played at a relaxing volume. Yes, sometimes blaring heavy metal can do the trick, but for the purposes of relaxation, it should be at a relaxing, soft level.

Music works well especially when it is predominantly instrumental. However, a pleasant voice can be equally effective. It is really up to you. Whatever you like, and what actually works.

Concentrate on the lyrics, or the instruments being played. Soak in the rhythm, the beats, the pace of the music. Let it flow over you, through you.

Sounds, especially those from nature, can be the most effective for relaxation, but some may make you want to dose off. Crickets, or frogs can do that, their soothing tones are a very effective means to drift off into slumber, but that is not the point of meditation after all.

Sounds of running water seems to make many people want to pee. Though not for me, but I can understand this situation. I have always preferred sounds from tropical forests, and these can often include thunderstorms, another favorite of mine, or even waterfalls or streams, but mostly tropical bird calls.

I employ tropical rainforest sounds especially in the winter, where I am cooped up inside for long periods, it is cold, dark, and gloomy outside, and I just want it to be sunny and summer again.

Ocean sounds are also comforting to many people. The crash of surf on the shore seems to have a calming effect.

Actual sounds outside are better, but only if you can manage the good ones without the other noise pollution sources in this busy world.

Exercise and Physical Activity

Non-exertive exercise can be quite helpful. Though spending time in a gym or outside running or walking can help bleed off much tension, and aggression because you have the opportunity to redirect the negative into something positive.

With certain anxieties though, visiting a gym may be intimidating. Purchasing weights may be an option, but they can get expensive, and definitely will clutter up a considerable space in your living areas. Perhaps consider a multiple function exercise machine of sorts instead of free weights if possible. Alternatively, you may consider practicing Yoga. It is a way to develop strength and stamina if you are able to perform the physical aspects.

Physical exercise may not always be possible, with weather and location restrictions, physical disabilities and limitations, or for many other reasons.

However, I find that even a short walk can make a huge difference in attitude and feeling better. If there is bad weather, and if you are able, visit a shopping mall where you can walk around in a safe, climate controlled indoor environment, or a skyway in a busy city. If you are fortunate to live in rural areas, there may be biking and walking trails to follow. I know several people that part of their daily routine is to walk a certain amount of miles and they love it.

For those of us with disabilities, even walking can be a challenge, so try to find substitutes that you are capable of. You don't need the expense of a gym, you can lift weights made from regular household items, like putting sand or rocks in a milk jug, or doing simple stretching and mobility exercises as you sit or stand. Depending upon your limitations, you may require assistance with even simple things, but the possibilities are there. Be creative, as any effort is going to be far better than no effort. Any amount of movement will be far better than no movement at all.

If you have the means to, take up swimming. This may even work out better for you if you have limiting disabilities. Being in the water can also be soothing, relaxing, and therapeutic.

Get a massage if you are able. This inherently removes the tensions from your physical being, and trust me, it is nearly impossible then for you to retain any bad sensations or thoughts after a good massage.

Take a nap if you can. Some may recommend against trying to sleep while experiencing strong emotions, but in reality that is probably the best time to try. You must relax, diffuse the tensions, and release strong emotions in order to drift off to sleep.

I do understand that some people may not have the physical ability to exercise in any way at all.

This is where the visual comes in.

Visual Aides

We mostly perceive the world through our eyes, and I don't mean to be offensive or inconsiderate in any way to the visually impaired.

Read a book, especially one that opens up your mind, and makes you think, or at least visualize the scenes described in the text. Reading comics can help also by invoking humor. You could read anything that you desire, even begin to learn new things while doing so, also a great benefit in the end. As long as it distracts you from the main problem.

Visual doesn't always include the use of your eyes. You can imagine a great many things with your mind.

Internally visualizing things can be a great way to distract your mind from negative thoughts and tendencies.

Even if you have never tried this, it is easy to learn, and practice virtually anywhere you are or go.

Among the visual effects you might enjoy is the use of lighting effects. In this, the possibilities are nearly endless. I like lighting that simulates being under water, and shimmering through the depths. A kaleidoscope casting dancing patterns and colors around the room has a very calming effect.

Aquariums can offer a lot of relaxation possibilities, just watching the little swimmers do their thing. However, the drawback here is that fish tanks can require a fair amount of maintenance.

Hobbies and Distractions

Hobbies often offer a great deal of relaxation, personal sense of well-being and even achievement, as well as a possible aesthetic and creative outlet. Not all hobbies can be accomplished well with physical limitations though, but there are a few that are manageable.

A hobby can be a collection of things, arts and crafts, knitting and other textile related endeavors; even bird watching can be considered a hobby. Gardening also offers the added benefit of seeing things grow, and also will help a bit on the grocery list expenses.

The point of any hobby is to distract you from problematic things, events, and situations that are causing difficulties, and adversity. The key to this being a 'distraction'. A positive means to remove or reduce the negative.

A hobby is also supposed to be considered enjoyable. If you are attempting anything that fosters or ends in frustration, anger, disappointment, or other negative results, then you are missing the point entirely, and should reconsider your efforts or particular hobby.

Find something that you can actually do, and then just do it. It doesn't even have to cost you anything other than time in some cases. There are even hobbies that you can do with or share with family and friends, as long as the endeavor accomplishes some relaxation, pleasure, and most importantly a sense of well-being.

Humor and Laughter

An additional effective method is the healing power of laughter. Sometimes it just eases the tension in ways no other method can manage.

Caution must be taken when employing this method though, as humor can easily become sarcastic, condescending, or even hurtful if used as a tool to vent anger inappropriately.

Joviality is good for the soul, and a good hearty belly laugh can be infectious. Of course, you should really have a very good reason for laughing in public or around other people, otherwise they may take it the wrong way and have you hauled away and locked up.

The same goes for maniacal laughter, though it does have its places and uses, it would not be a good idea to give off an impression that you are an evil mad-scientist after all.

You can find humor in all sorts of places, like people watching. This can be entertaining in all manner of ways.

Clumsiness, dating ritual failures, food mishaps, or even wardrobe mishaps, and watching people generally not paying attention when walking around. Learn to play games while out watching others, see if you can identify potential disaster victims before they happen.

Above all, have fun, let that frustration go, and replace it with humor and laughter.

Social Interaction

Friends are great, and if you have any, spend some time with them. Just hanging out, talking, whatever. If they are a good friend, they will listen to you. Don't make your problems the only subject you ever talk about though, this gets very tedious for the listener.

Make conversations interesting, show interest in what your friend or friends have to say, ask about how they are and listen to them.

Bring up certain sensitive subjects anonymously if possible. For instance, say something like you have this other friend or know someone else who is thinking of something or whatever to get their feedback on the subject. Talk things out, you will feel better.

I know a lot of people that have a lot of difficulty in this area. They need to talk, but just can't bring themselves around to doing so. If you find yourself in the presence of anyone like this, extend to them an open invitation to be there for them and listen, should they decide to open up. Don't make them open up. Let them make that decision on their own. If they feel they can trust you, they will.

If anything, convey the fact that you are no different than they, that we all have things we need to get off our chests in life, and it is good to do so. Keeping things bottled up only lead to long-term problems.

Natural Surroundings

Being outside on a perfect, sunny, summer day is the best possible experience you could ever find. Nothing quite like being out in nature, no traffic, no people, no construction, no aircraft, just you and nature.

Parks are excellent for this experience, but some charge fees, and often there are other people around as well, not to mention pets. If you have the means, and the time, find a nice natural preserve somewhere where you can go off and spend some 'alone' time with nature.

A deserted beach works as well, but a forest is nice also.

Sensory deprivation / Overload

Ah, the senses. We deal with them all the time, unless you have some impairment in life, deafness, blindness, etc... and taking a break from these senses can be an interesting experience. Nothing outside of the body interferes with the inner workings and thoughts of the mind in a sensory deprivation tank. Designed to relieve the occupant of all light, sounds, and smells, you are suspended in a comfortable temperature water compartment. Free to float in silence, and darkness. Nothing to cause your mind to be distracted.

If you cannot relax under these conditions, nothing will help you.

Sensory overload is the diametric opposite of deprivation, where all your active senses are overwhelmed simultaneously. This has a desensitizing effect on them, much like how your ears will ring after attending a live concert, or being temporarily blinded by a bright light source. This particular practice does carry with it some risk of damaging your senses, or at least impairing them for a time. I would not recommend it.

Ongoing Efforts and Management

Managing diabetes is going to be a full-time occupation for some, and with diligence, determination, and help, it can be overcome entirely or at the very least, managed.

Stick to a better diet, relax, and use every opportunity to dispel the effects of diabetes. Moods can be manipulated, especially by external positive sources, so find these as often as possible and frequently revisit them.

Diabetes doesn't have to ruin your life, work or relationships. Take it back no matter how futile it may seem at times, there is always a better way to feel and live.

You have to understand that not every situation has an amicable resolution, that some things just are the way they are, and nothing you can do, no matter how angry or frustrated you are, will ever change that. Accept it for what it is. Accept it as part of life, and learn how to let things go.

Many say that diabetes is irreversible, and they will push upon you medications for this or that symptom. I contend that if you exercise adequately, eat sensibly, and maintain a strict elimination of the foods harming you, in the end, diabetes can be not only controlled, but almost entirely taken out of your life.

As mentioned earlier, you may or may not really care about your own health, but consider the added burden you will place on your spouse and family if you succumb to the effects of diabetes. You really don't want to lose a foot, or a leg, you really don't want to depend upon a cane, walker or wheelchair to get around. They are useful, but they suck having to use anywhere because in spite of the American Disability Association requirements by law, they are always a last consideration by most Architects and Civil Engineers. I know this from experience.

It is not fun having to depend upon anyone else to help you get around, change your clothing, bathe, eat, sleep, or use the lavatory.

It is a simple matter really to take control of your life, your diet, and your health to ensure that you stay happy, healthy, mobile and active in life. Don't give in to despair or depression, this is not incurable and can be prevented altogether. Had I known earlier in life what I now know, I probably never would have even developed diabetes, and my father might still be alive today, and diabetes free also.

You owe it to everyone around you and loves you to fix this problem, or prevent it in the first place.

Author's Note:

I thank you for your patronage and hope that you enjoy your new book! Reviews are encouraged; please feel free to share your experience with others.

~Kevin R. Sweeter

Follow on my Amazon Author Page: https://www.amazon.com/Kevin-R.Sweeter/e/B00500O7U4

Keep up to date with availability and promotions.

Contact E-mail: kevin.sweeter.author@gmail.com

Please subscribe to my author email list for news, updates, and special offers and events.

Like, Follow, and Share on my Facebook Author Page: https://www.facebook.com/Kevin-Sweeter-Author-209756967060/

Visit the book pages; see what is in the works, what is published, what will come soon, and what the books are about. Invite your friends to 'like' my pages.